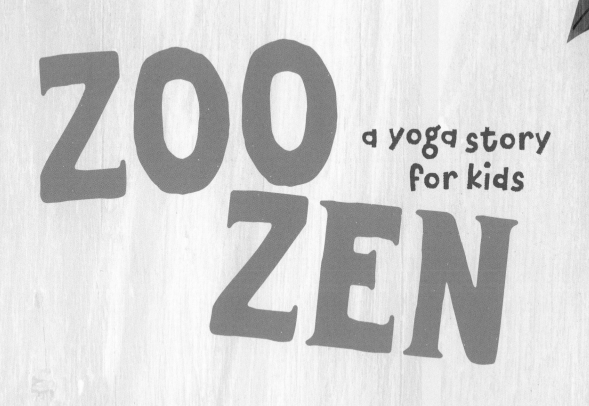

ZOO
ZEN

a yoga story for kids

Kristen Fischer

illustrated by
Susi Schaefer

sounds true
BOULDER, COLORADO

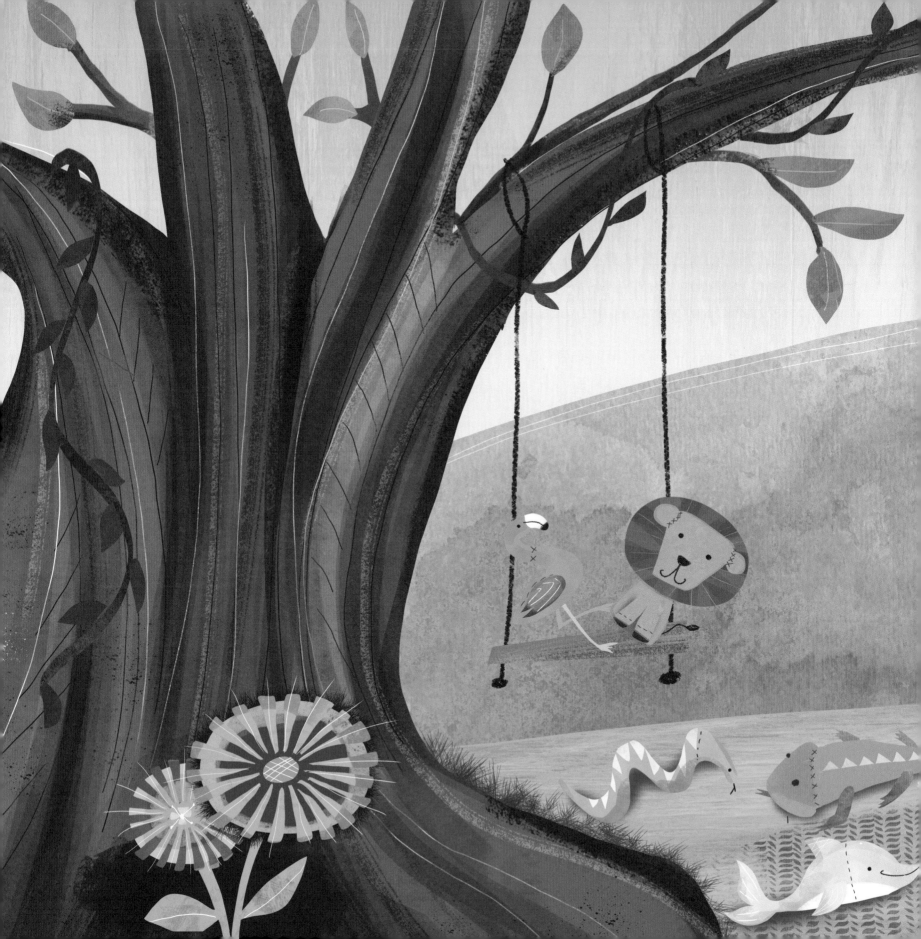

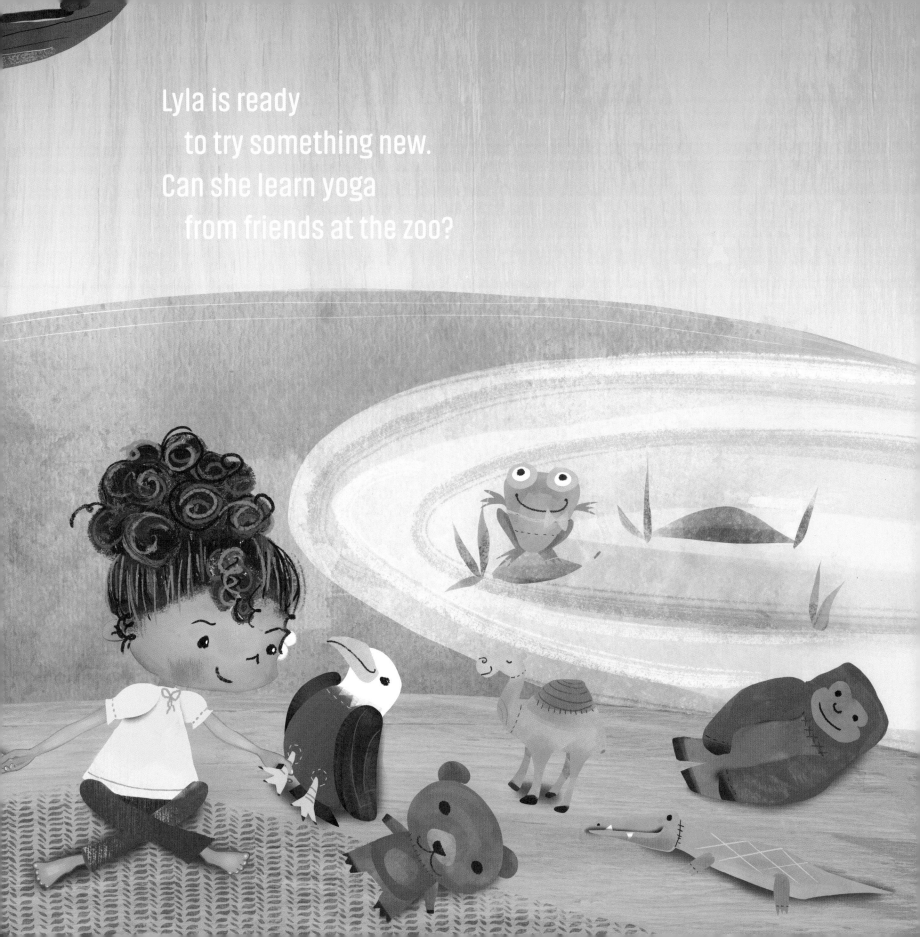

Lyla is ready
    to try something new.
Can she learn yoga
    from friends at the zoo?

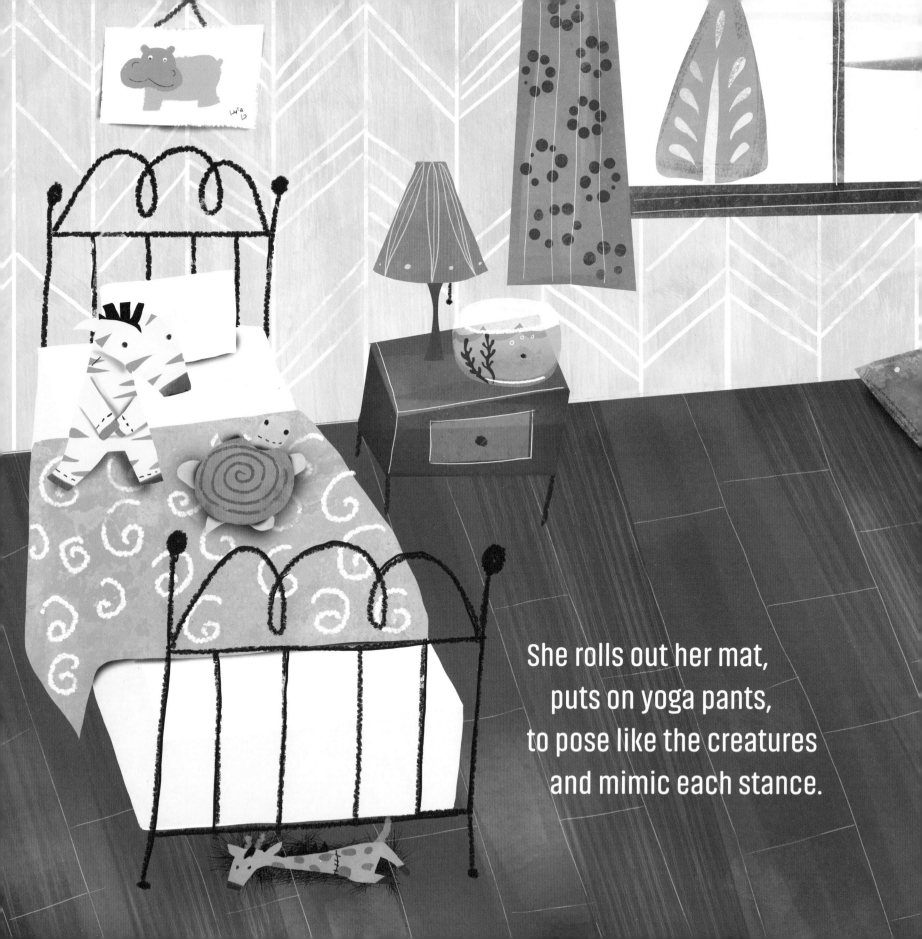

She rolls out her mat,
puts on yoga pants,
to pose like the creatures
and mimic each stance.

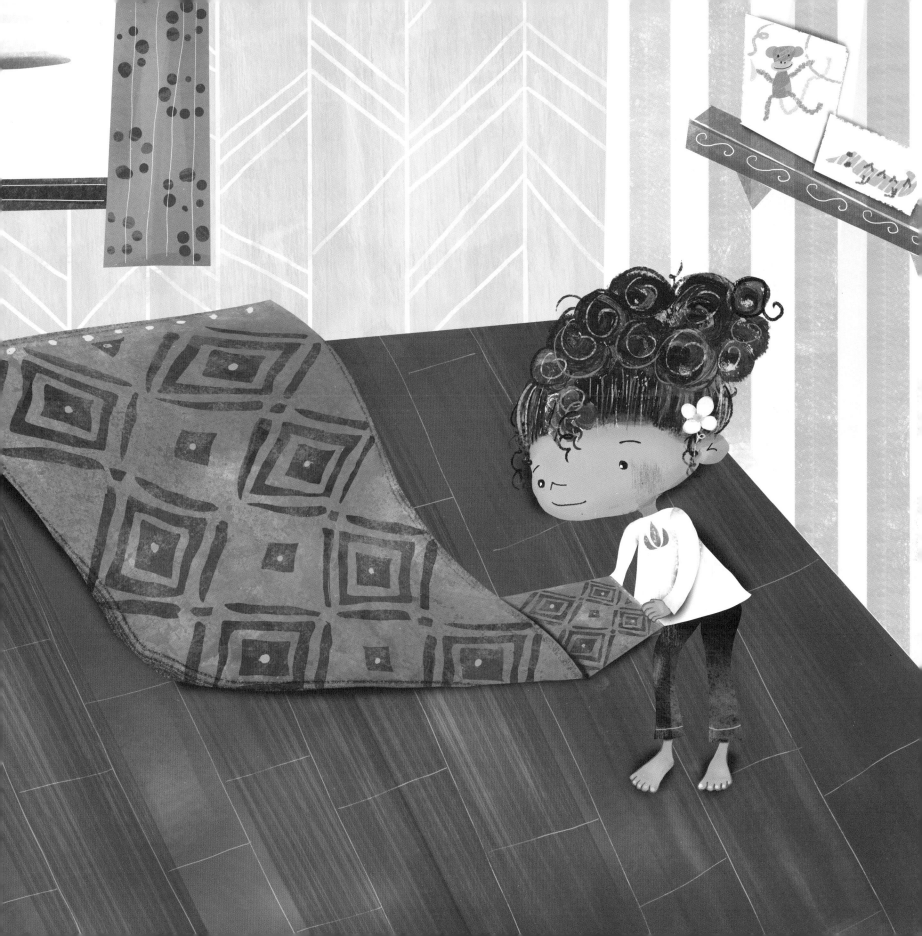

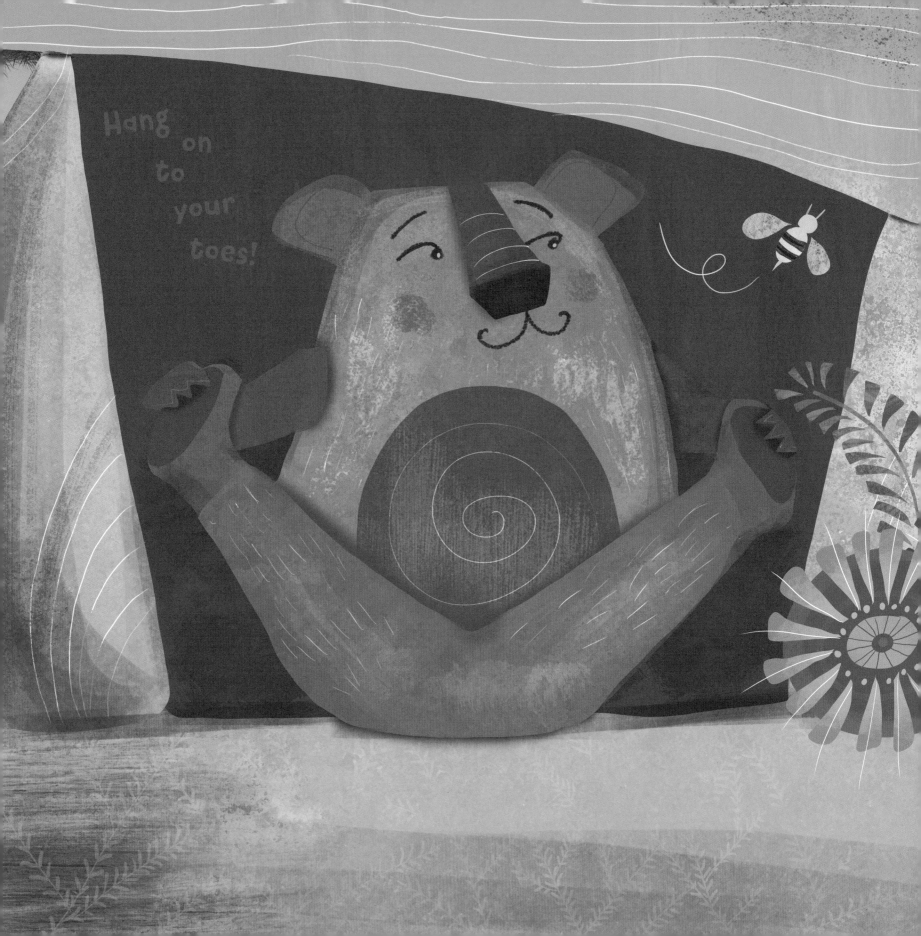

Hang on to your toes!

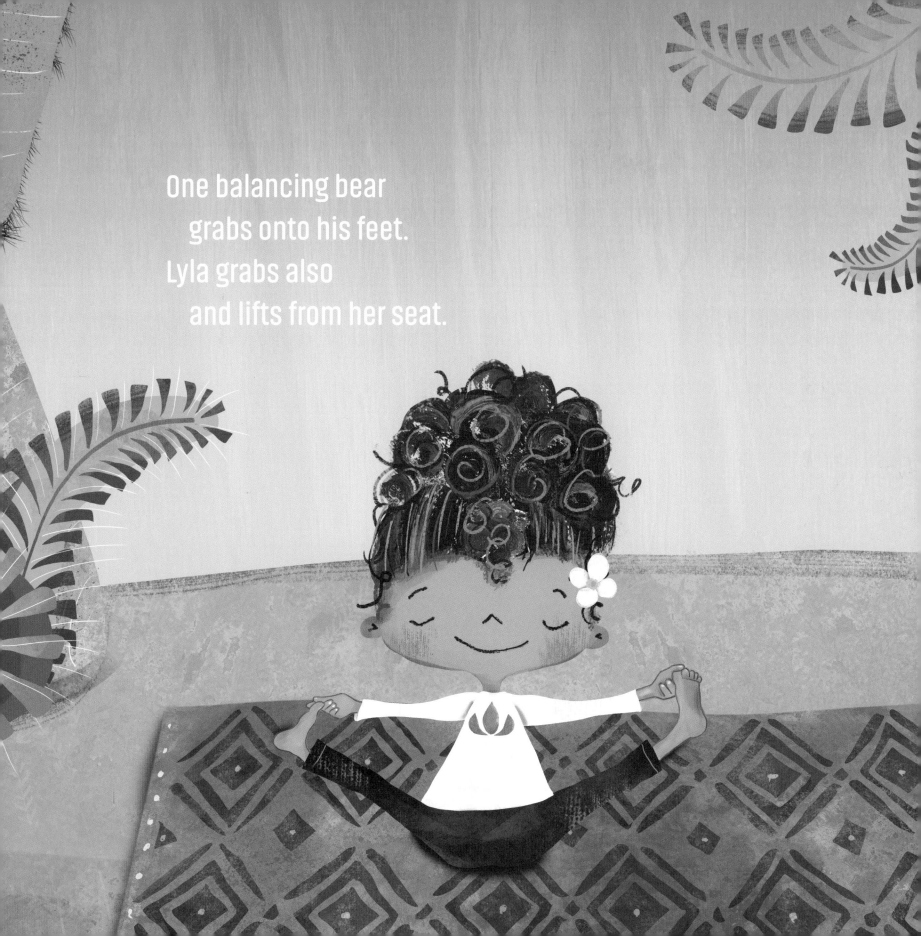

One balancing bear
grabs onto his feet.
Lyla grabs also
and lifts from her seat.

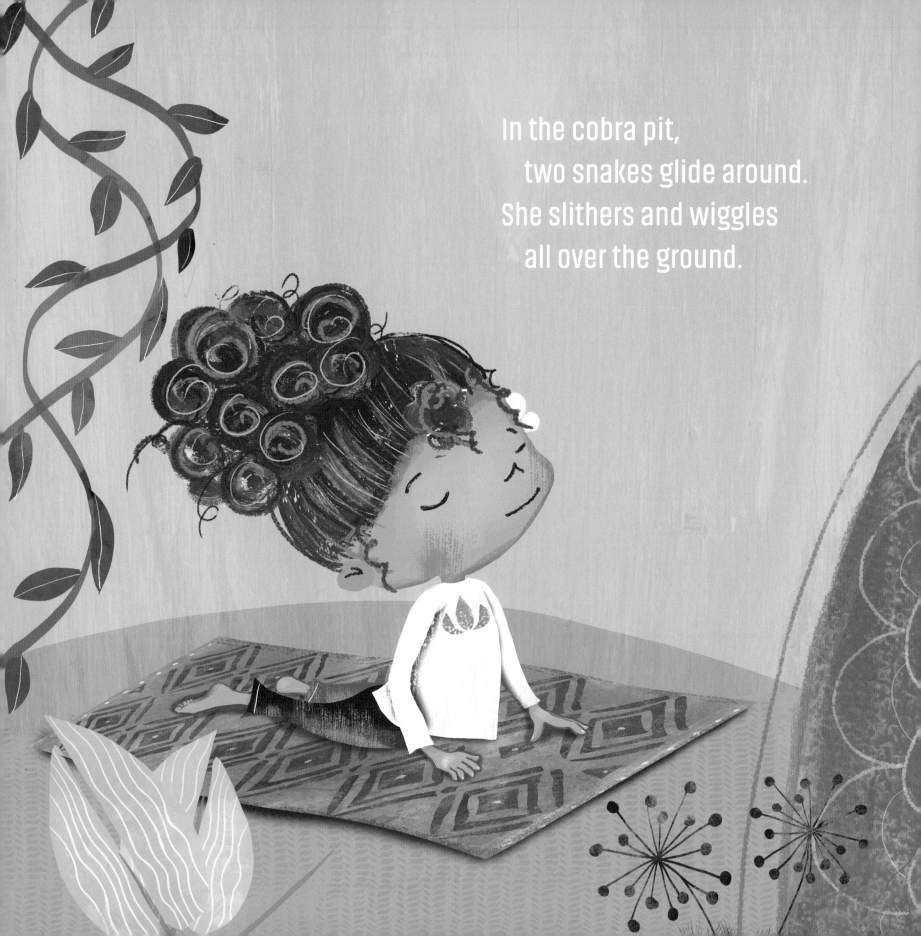

In the cobra pit,
two snakes glide around.
She slithers and wiggles
all over the ground.

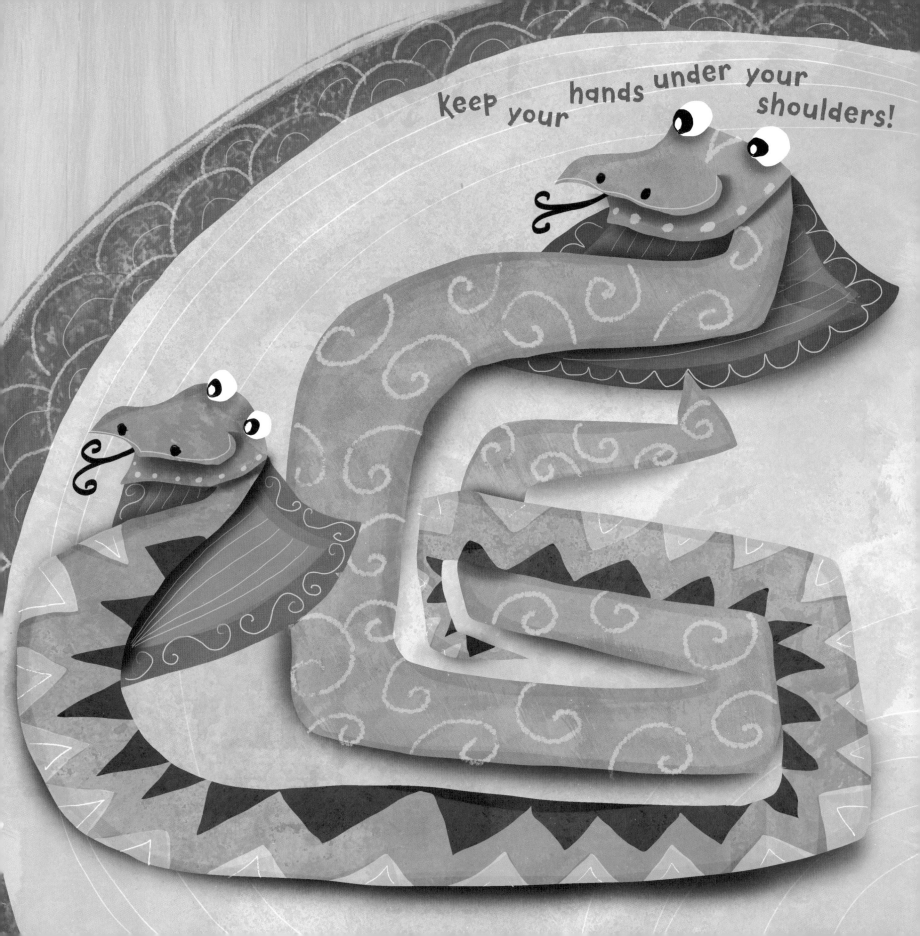

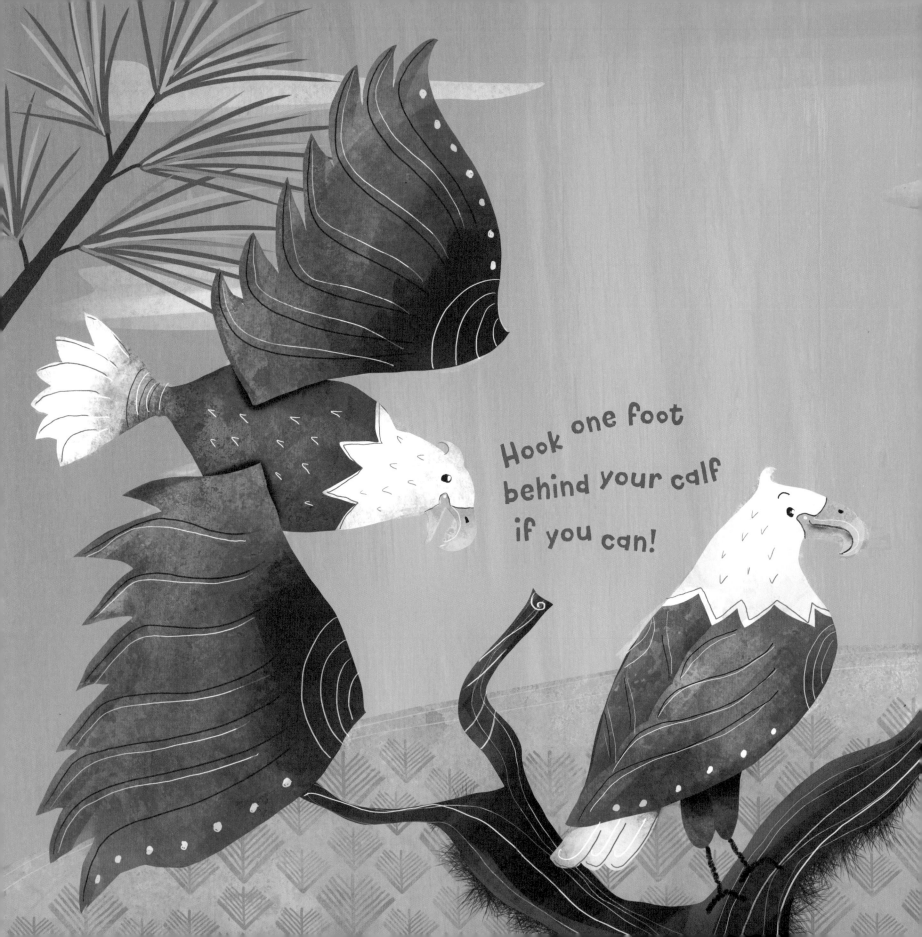

Hook one foot
behind your calf
if you can!

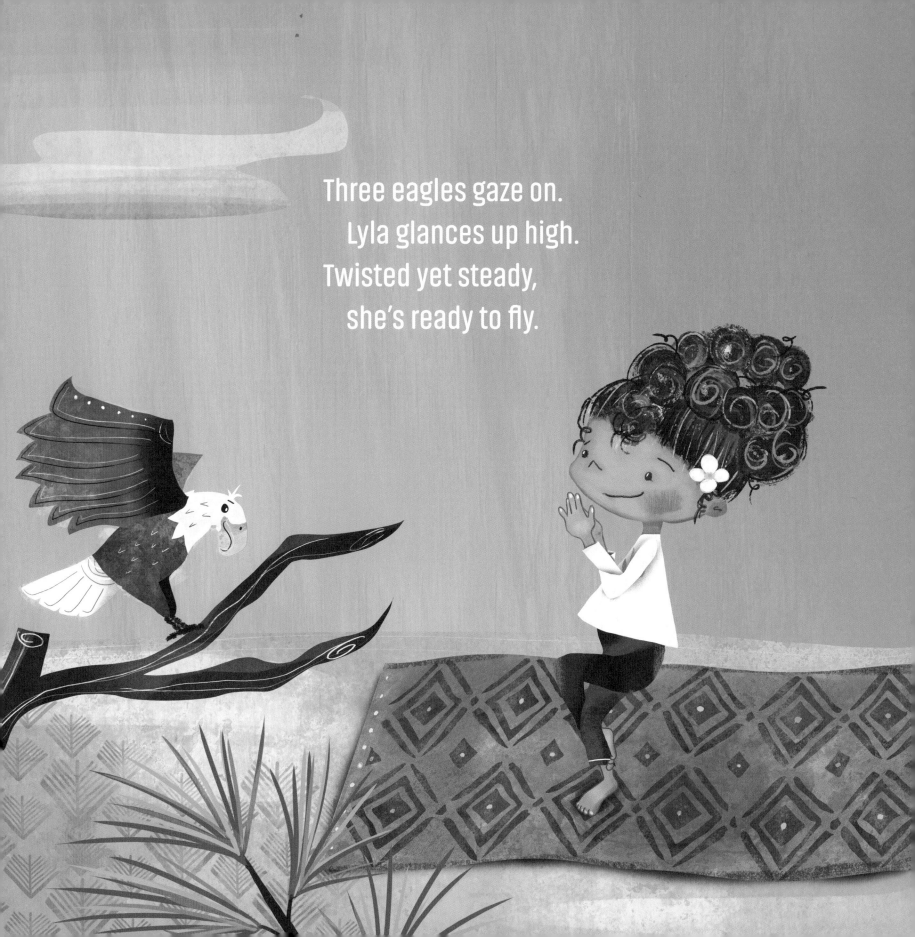

Three eagles gaze on.
Lyla glances up high.
Twisted yet steady,
she's ready to fly.

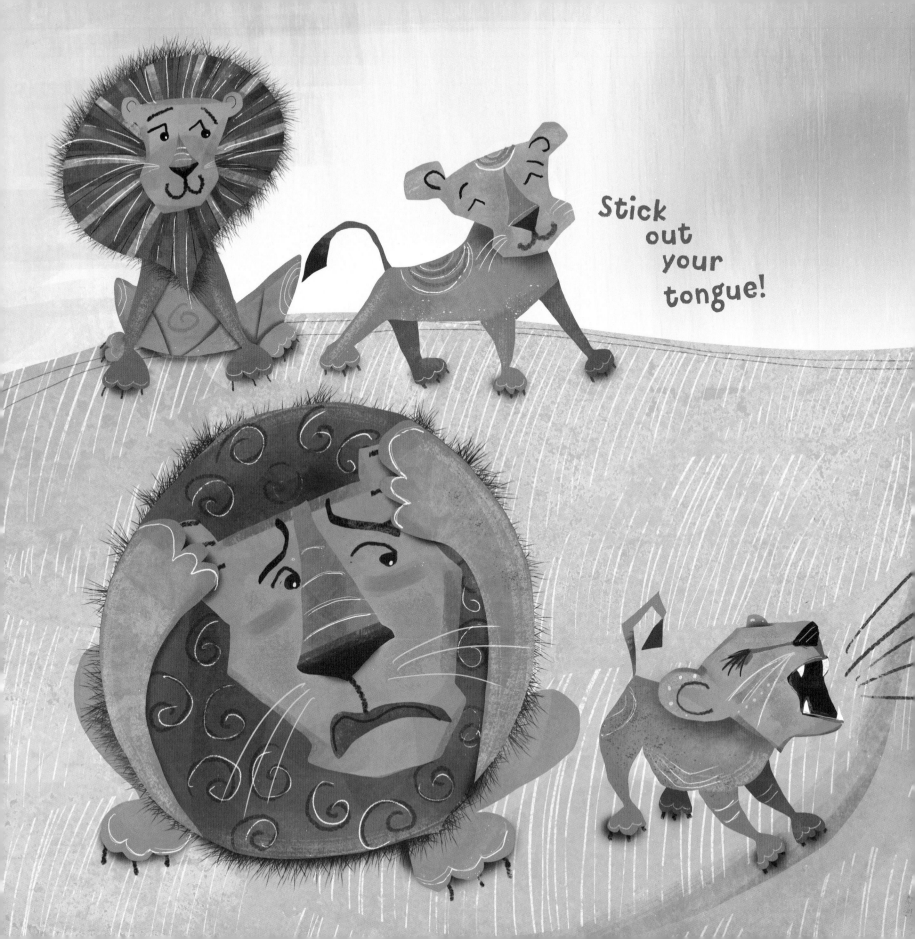

Stick
out
your
tongue!

Lions stalk and they prowl,
in this pride there are four.
Hands pressed to her knees,
Lyla bellows a roar.

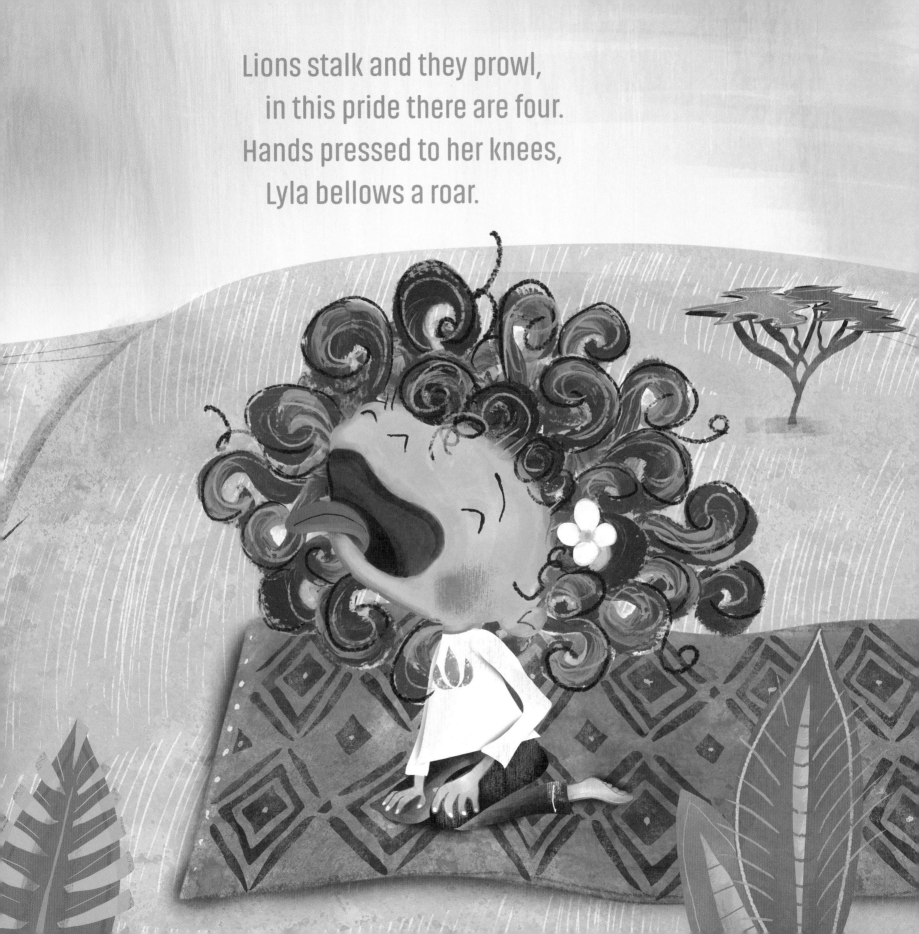

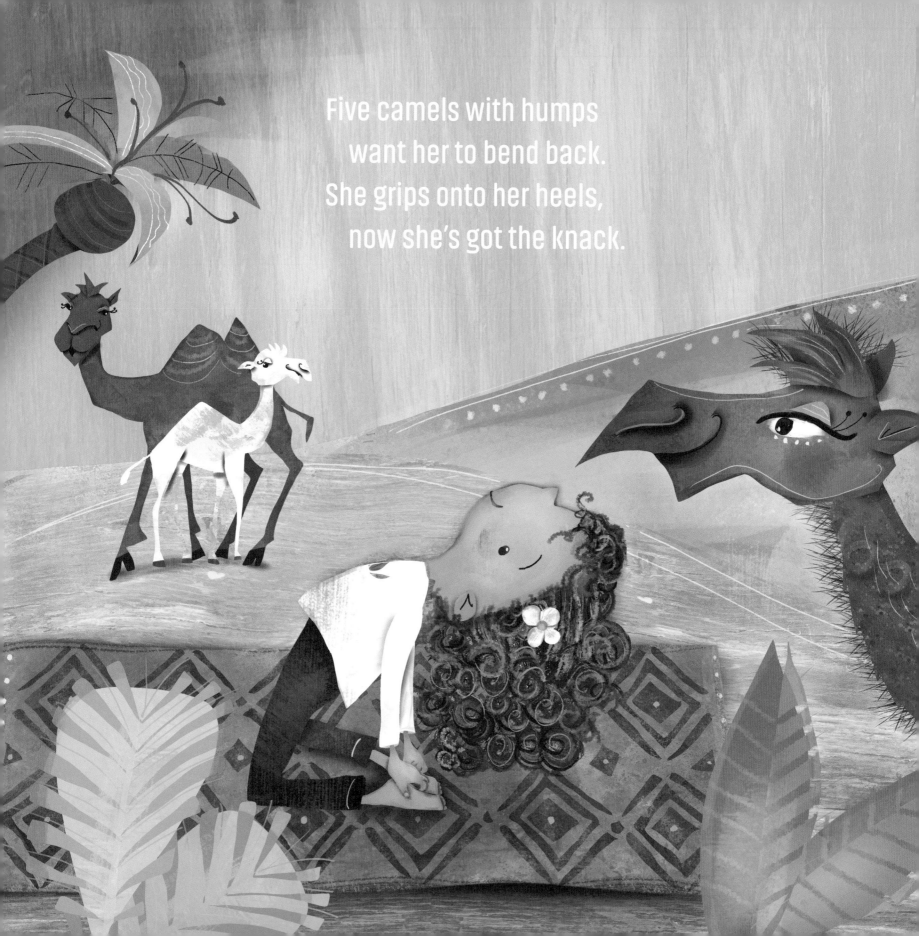

Five camels with humps
want her to bend back.
She grips onto her heels,
now she's got the knack.

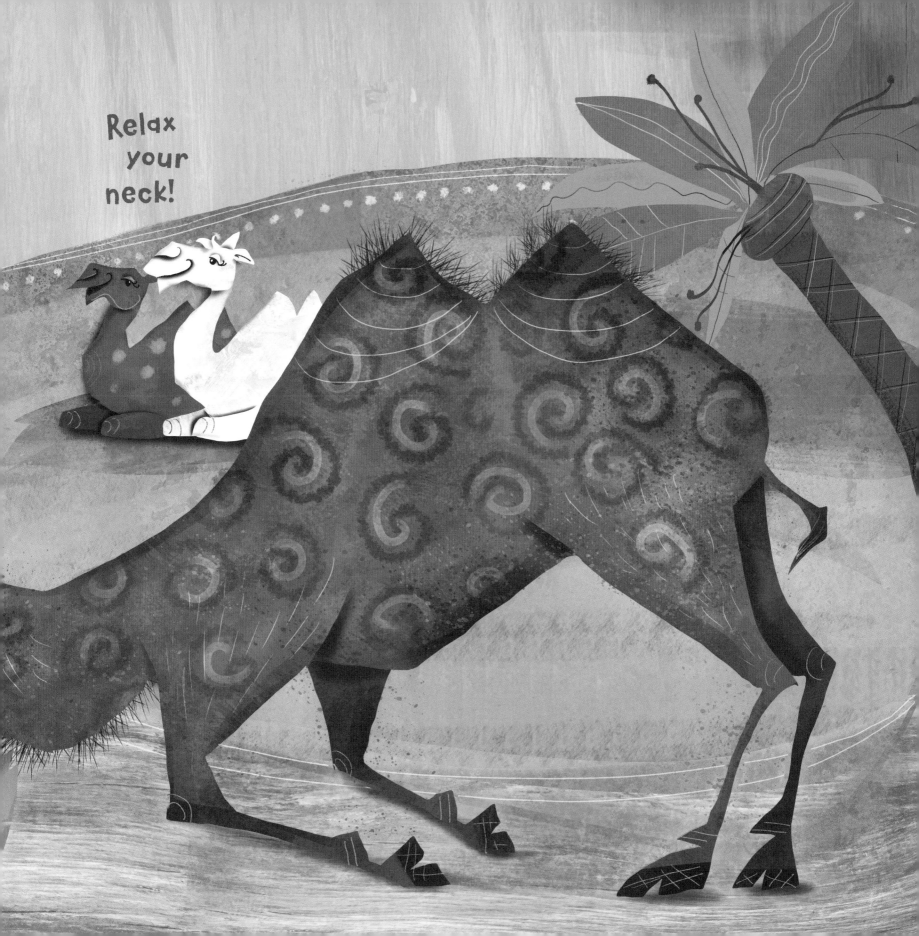

Like six crocodiles
    perched up on their claws,
she's on her tummy
    and makes time to pause.

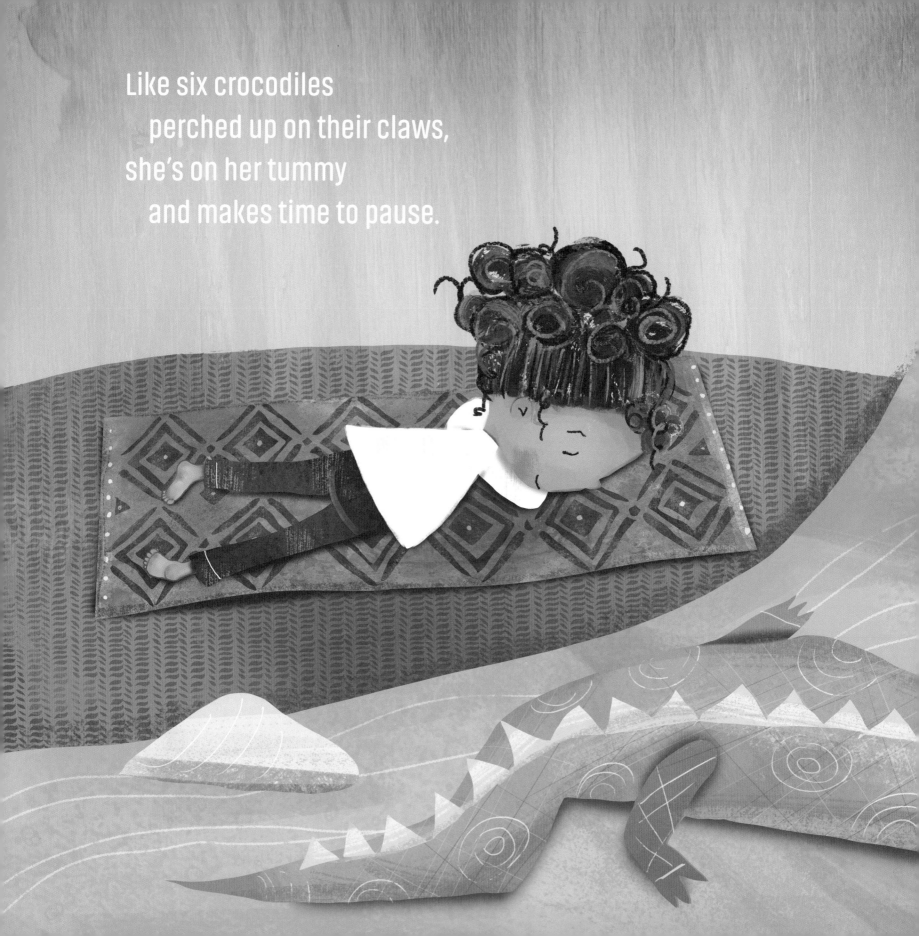

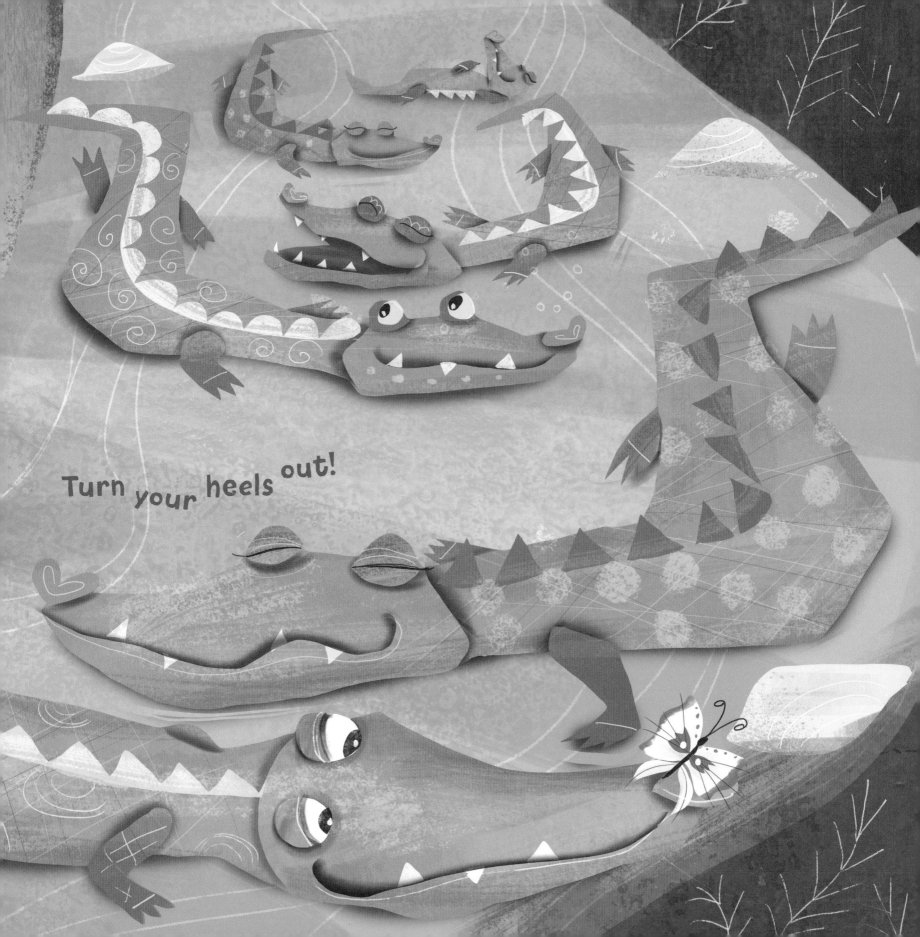

Turn your heels out!

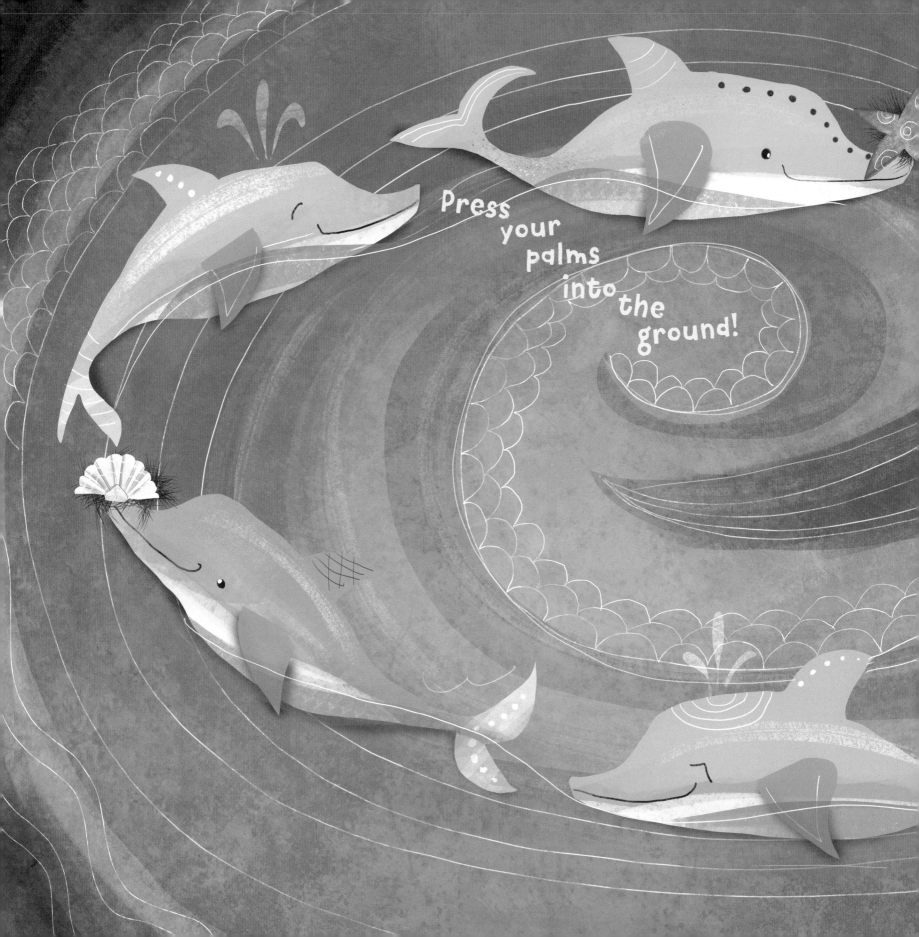

Press your palms into the ground!

Seven dolphins arrive
and swim close to her mat.
Raising her bottom,
her forearms stay flat.

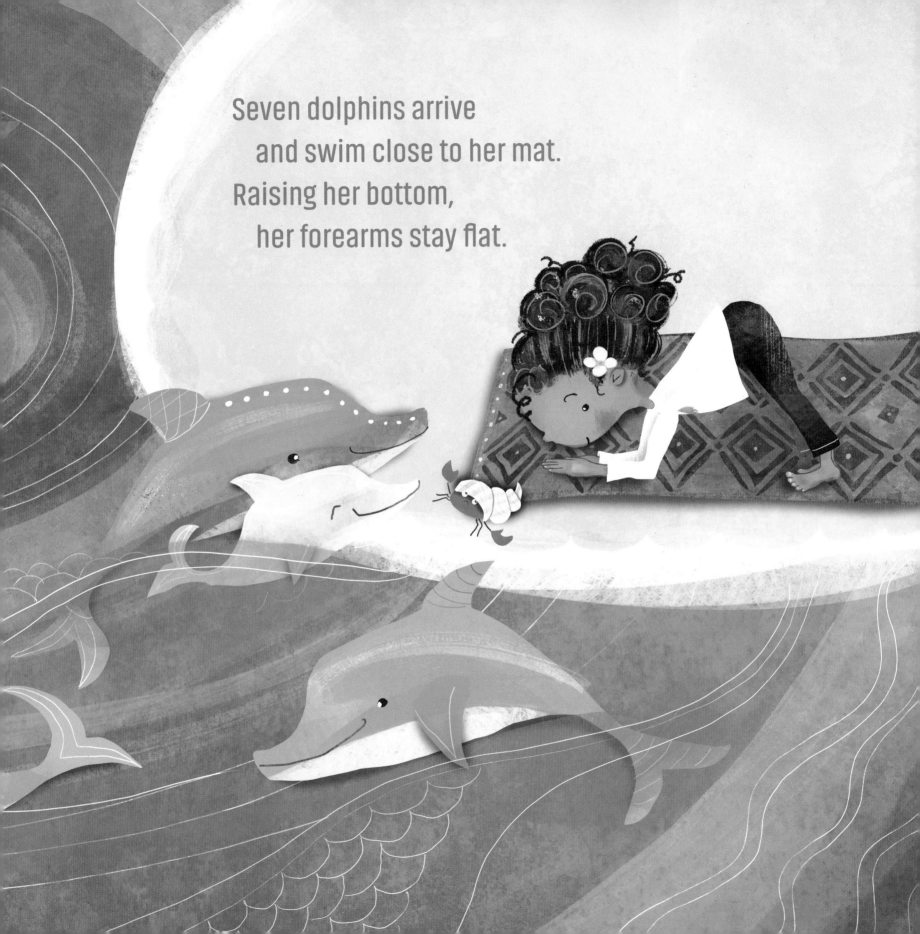

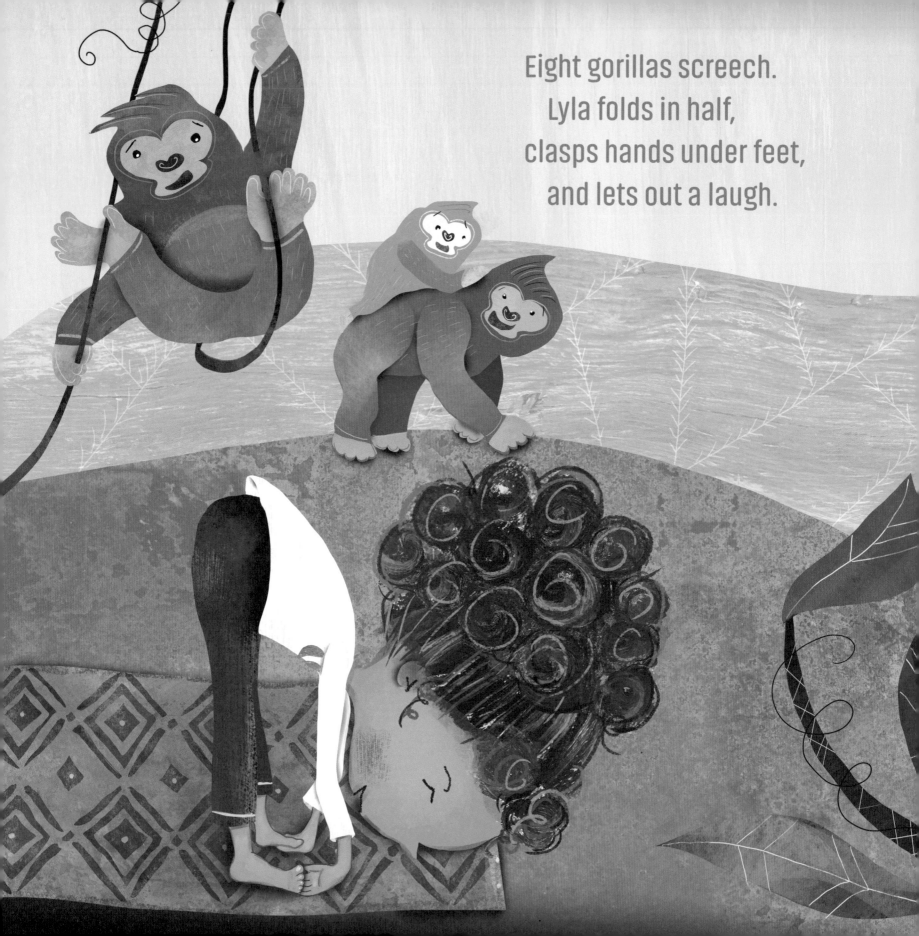

Eight gorillas screech.
Lyla folds in half,
clasps hands under feet,
and lets out a laugh.

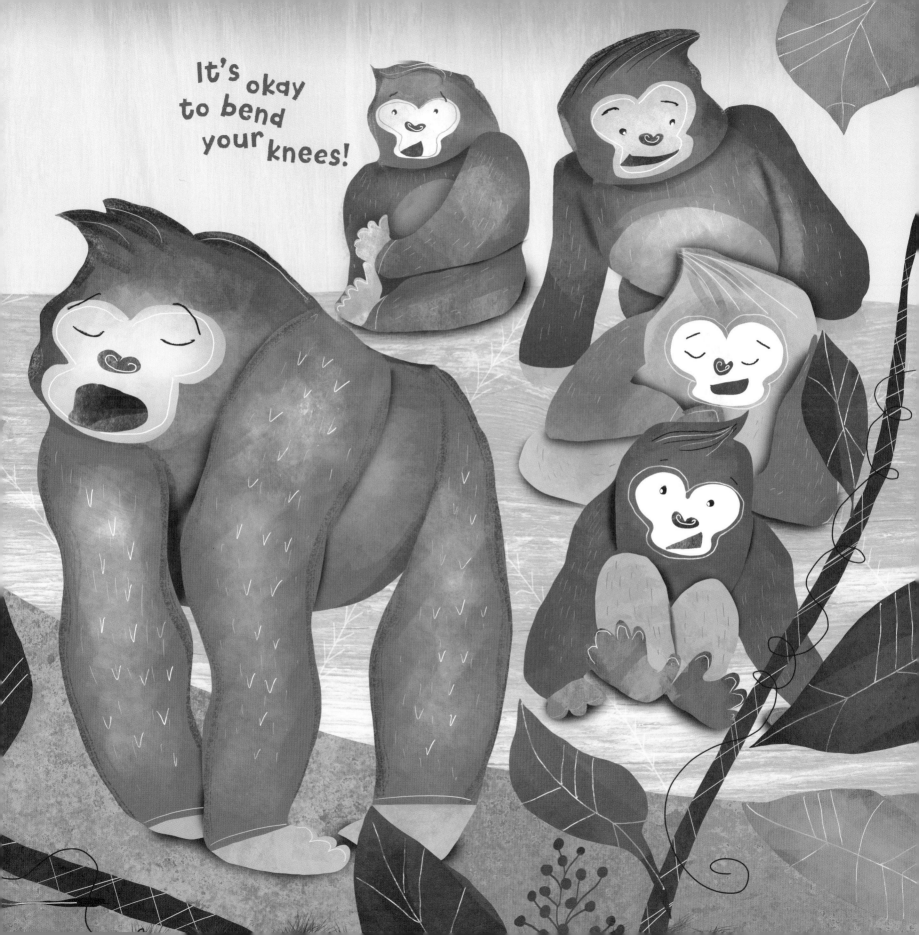

Nine scaly lizards
    climb onto a stone.
Her leg is a tail
    she's only just grown.

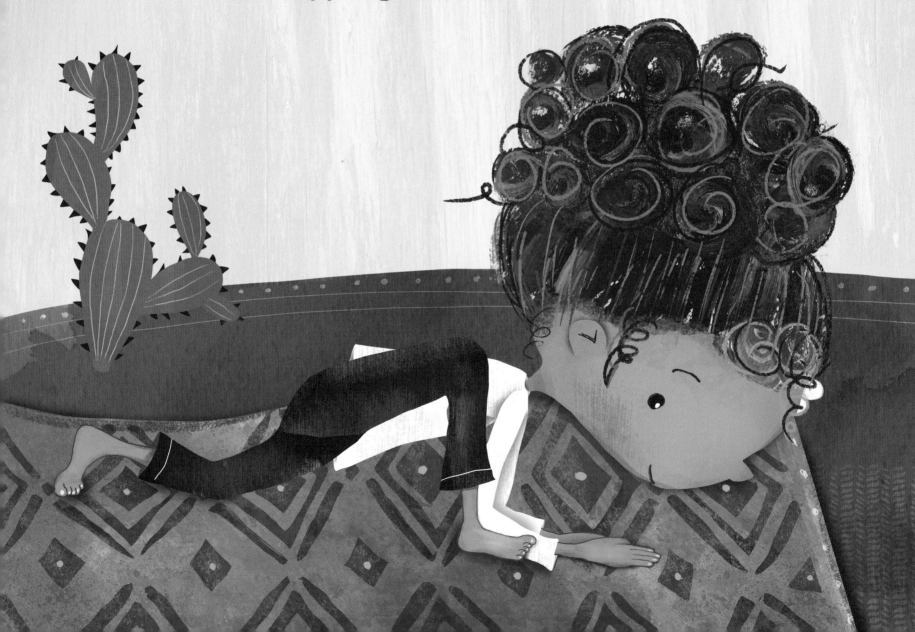

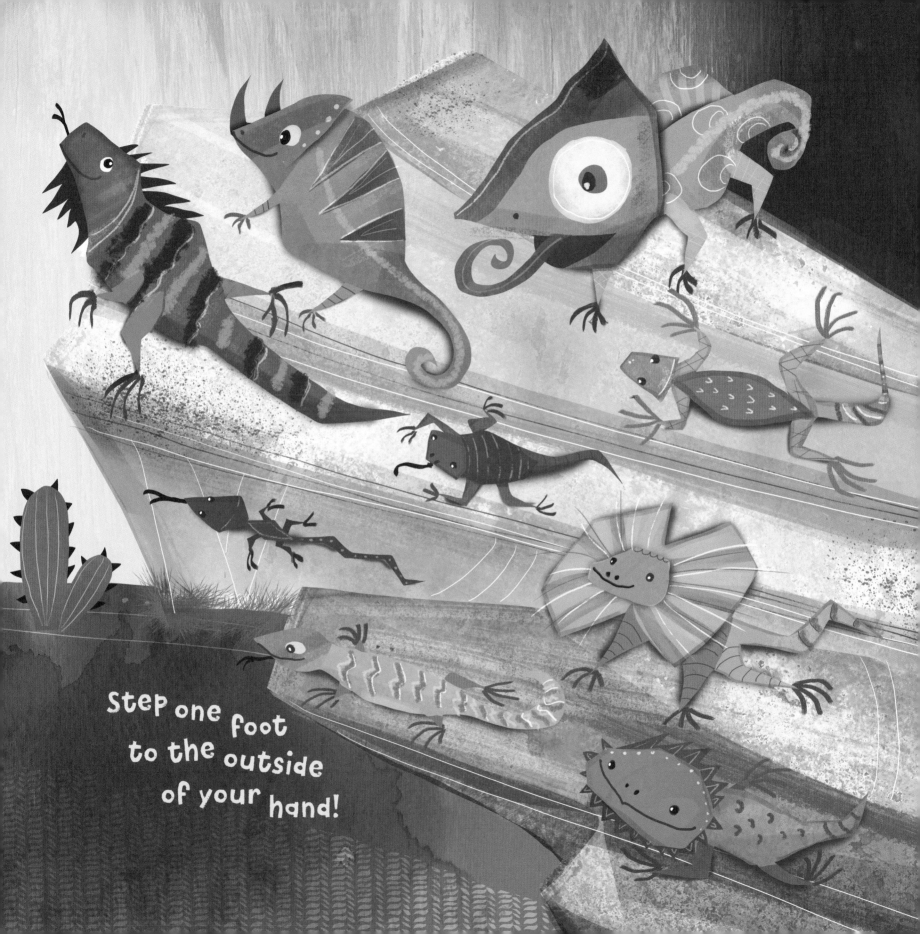

Step one foot
to the outside
of your hand!

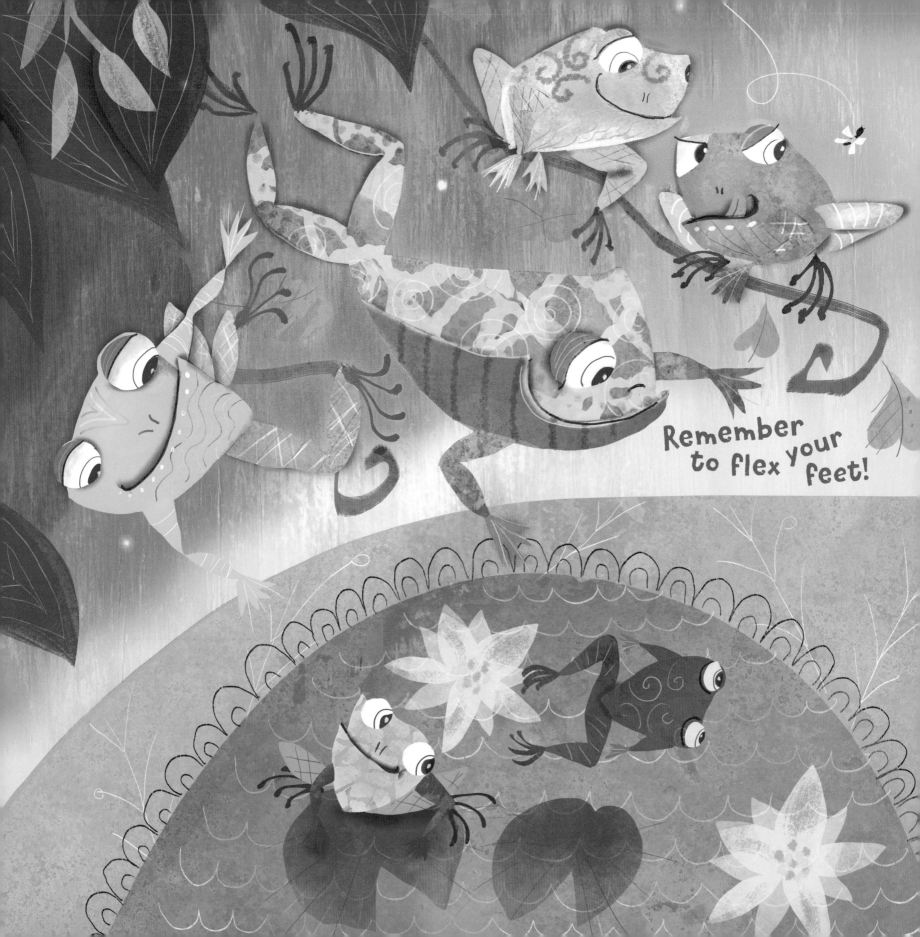

Remember to flex your feet!

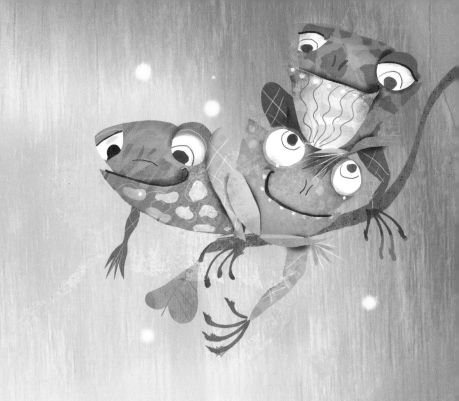

Ten frogs by a pond,
some hip and some hop.
She stretches out wide,
her arms are the prop.

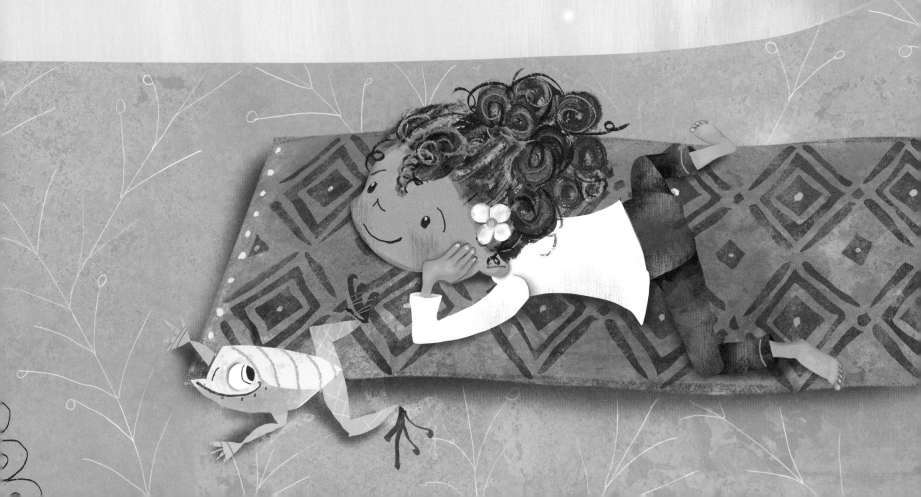

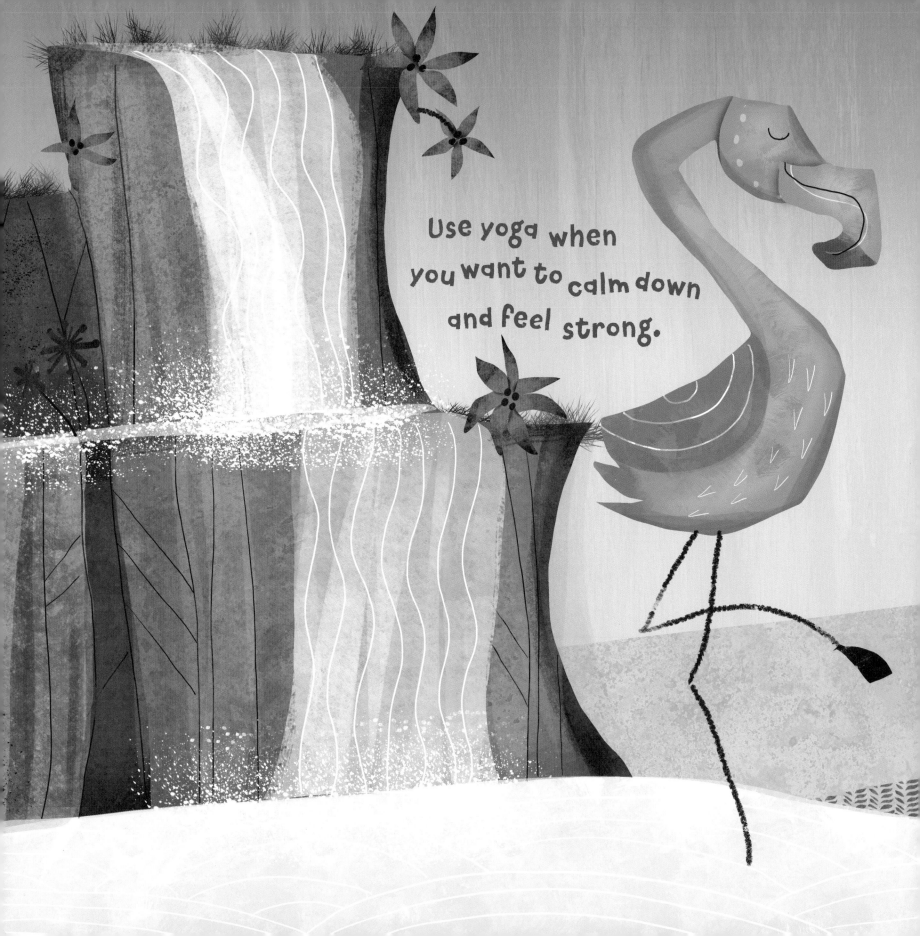

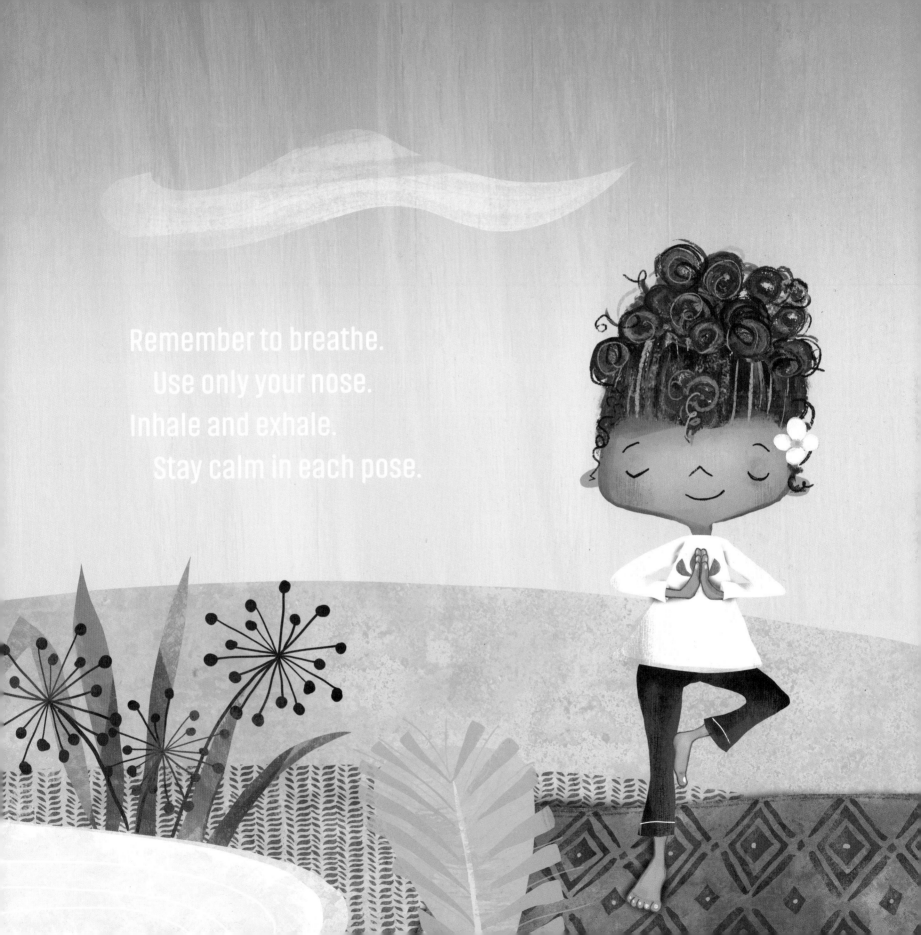

Remember to breathe.
Use only your nose.
Inhale and exhale.
Stay calm in each pose.

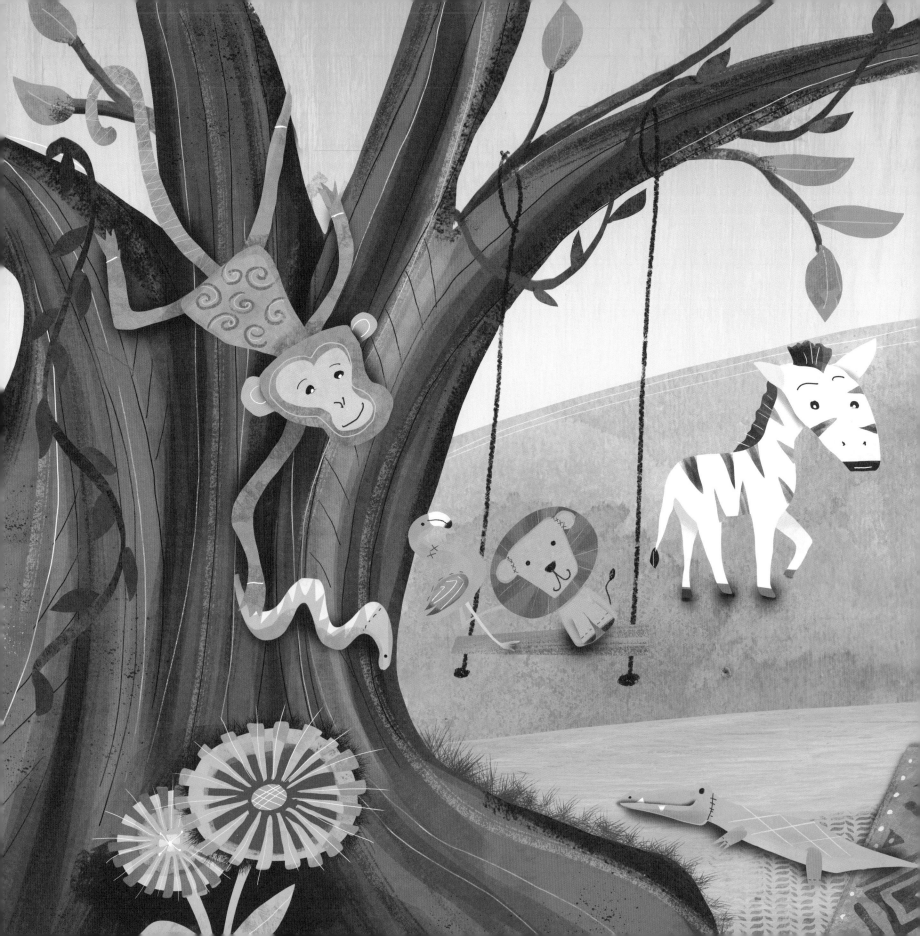

Always be present,
right here and right now.
Show that you're thankful.
Conclude with a bow.

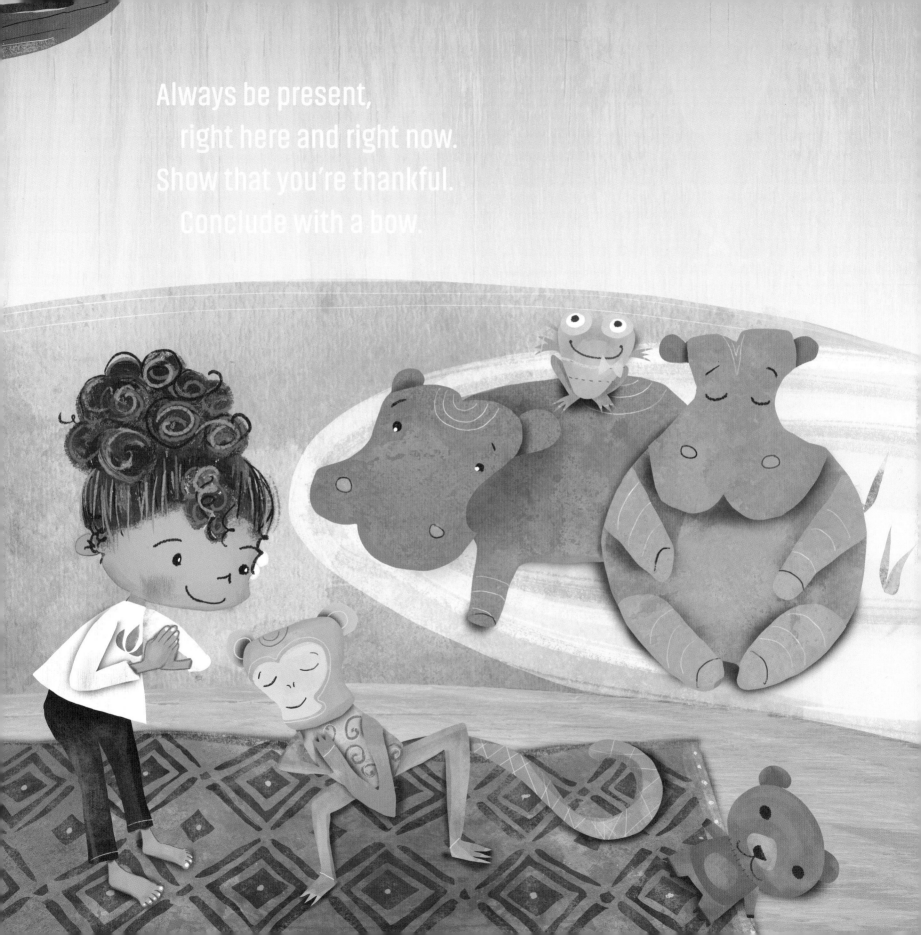

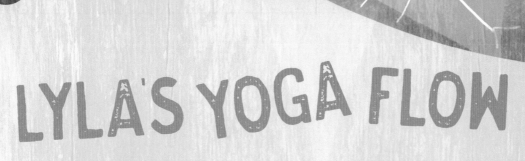

LYLA'S YOGA FLOW

Begin Lyla's yoga flow in a cross-legged pose with your hands resting on your thighs. Breathe in and out of your nose.

1. Bear Pose

Sit up with the soles of your feet together. Grab your big toes and sit back to balance on your bottom. Slowly extend your legs straight as you gaze up and continue breathing.

2. Cobra Pose

Lie face down on a mat with your legs behind you. Press the tops of your feet into the mat. Place your hands under your shoulders. Next, breathe in as you gently lift your head and chest off the mat. Straighten your arms as much as possible, keeping elbows close to the sides of your body. Continue to breathe as you hold the pose. Then breathe out as you lower yourself down to the mat.

3. Eagle Pose

Stand up with your feet just a little apart. Bend your knees. Lift up your left leg and balance on your right foot. Now cross your left thigh over the right one, pointing your left toe down. Hook your toes behind your right calf, if you can. Stretch your arms out in front of you, and cross your right arm over your left. Bend your elbows and press the backs of your hands together. Gaze upwards as you breathe.

4. Lion Pose

Kneel on a mat and sit back on your heels. Press your palms into your knees, splaying out your fingers like claws. As you breathe in through your nose, open your mouth and try to stretch your tongue to your chin. Breathe out through your mouth and let out a roar!

5. Camel Pose

Kneel down on a mat. Sit up tall so your shins press into the mat. Place the palms of your hands on your back, just above your bottom, with fingers pointing down. Breathe in and arch your back, pressing your shoulder blades together. Keep your head up. Reach your right hand back and try to grab your heel. See if you can reach your left hand back to your left heel too. Breathe.

6. Crocodile Pose

On a mat, lie on your belly, cross your arms under your head and rest your forehead on your wrists. Relax into the mat and let your heels turn out. Breathe.

7. Dolphin Pose

Get onto your hands and knees on a mat with your knees below your hips. Put your forearms on the mat. Press your palms into the mat. Step up on your toes and lift your knees away from the mat, keeping them slightly bent. Lift your bottom to the sky. Let your head stay facing down.

8. Gorilla Pose

Stand up and fold at your hips, so your knees reach your toes. It's okay to bend your knees a little. Lift up your toes and slide your hands under them, palms up, fingers parallel to your toes. Now your hands are under your feet. Breathe, focusing on lifting your hips to the sky.

9. Lizard Pose

Bring your palms to the ground and extend your legs back, raising your bottom up and hanging your head. Place your right foot to the right of your pinky finger. Be sure your right knee is directly above your heel and not in front of it. For a deeper stretch, rest your forearms on the ground. Keep your chin lifted and look ahead.

10. Frog Pose

Come onto your hands and knees. Walk your knees out as wide as possible while still being comfortable. Bring your elbows and forearms to the ground beneath your shoulders. Keep palms flat on the ground.

11. Tree Pose

Stand up tall on a mat. Put your weight onto your left foot and lift your right foot off the mat. Place the sole of your right foot against the inside of your left leg, on your calf or above your knee. Place your hands together, palms touching, at the center of your chest. Breathe.

End Lyla's yoga flow by putting your hands together, palms touching, in the center of your chest. Bow and say *Namaste*, which means, "The light within me honors the light within you."

For Charlotte, Quinnan, Lyla, and Sydney—
my unexpected blessings.

Thank you for bringing
so much joy into my life.

K.F.

For Rich, Heidi, and Liam—
my cheerleaders at home.

For Brooks—my cheerleader
away from home.

For my parents—
my first cheerleaders ever.

S.S.

Sounds True
Boulder, CO 80306

Text © 2017 by Kristen Fischer
Illustrations © 2017 by Susi Schaefer

Cover and book design by Rachael Murray
Printed in South Korea

Library of Congress Cataloging-in-Publication Data
Names: Fischer, Kristen, author. | Schaefer, Susi, illustrator.
Title: Zoo zen : a yoga story for kids / by Kristen Fischer ; illustrated by Susi Schaefer.
Description: Boulder, CO : Sounds True, [2017] | Summary: Lyla learns yoga poses and gets some tips from the animals
    at the zoo as she observes one bear, two snakes, and more. Includes step-by-step instructions for doing each pose.
Identifiers: LCCN 2016047181 (print) | LCCN 2017004013 (ebook) | ISBN 9781622038916 (hardcover) |
    ISBN 1622038916 (hardcover) | ISBN 9781622039067 (ebook) | ISBN 1622039068 (ebook)
Subjects: | CYAC: Stories in rhyme. | Yoga—Fiction. | Zoo animals—Fiction. | Counting.
Classification: LCC PZ8.3.F62843 Zoo 2017 (print) | LCC PZ8.3.F62843 (ebook) | DDC [E—dc23
LC record available at https://lccn.loc.gov/2016047181

10 9 8 7 6 5 4 3 2 1